Midlife Musings
Creative Croning Ceremonies

June Hill

Order this book online at www.trafford.com
or email orders@trafford.com

Most Trafford titles are also available at major online book retailers.

OTHER CONTRIBUTORS:
      Edited by: Linda Griffin, Diane Meyers
      Contributors: Linda Griffin, Christy Morrell
      Photography by: iSTOCK

Print information available on the last page.

ISBN: 978-1-4251-2497-7 (sc)

Trafford rev. 07/16/2018

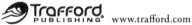 www.trafford.com

North America & international
toll-free: 1 888 232 4444 (USA & Canada)
fax: 812 355 4082

CONTENTS

Chapter 3

CELEBRATE YOUR CRONEHOOD

Chapter 4

CREATIVE WAYS TO CELEBRATE YOUR CRONEHOOD

AFTERTHOUGHT

FINAL THOUGHT

Dedication

To all crones and wisewomen who helped and inspired me to write this book, to my parents who had the courage to emigrate to the United States fifty years ago, to Bill, to my extended family of dear, close friends, and finally to my Corgi, Sophie, who is a source of joy in my life and always laughs at my jokes.

"Verily, great grace may go with a little gift; and precious are all things that come from friends."
—Theocritus

Introduction

My Dear Crone,

By my fiftieth birthday, I'd gone through that tunnel of fire called menopause without a gray hair on my head being scorched, thankfully. I felt a new source of energy that seemed to come out of nowhere; and I didn't know how, but I planned to spend the last phase of my life making a difference in the world! (But before I set out on that mission, I wanted to bring together several dear friends to open a bottle of champagne and rejoice!)

So I looked for unique ways to celebrate my post-menopausal triumph and started doing some research on rites of passage ceremonies. Through my research I saw words I hadn't seen before, like the *crone* and *croning ceremonies*, which I learned have their roots in ancient society. The crone is a woman who has gone through menopause and a croning ceremony is a spiritual, symbolic event that specifically honors a woman who has gone through that transition. Although I knew that becoming an elder is respected and revered in other cultures, when was the last time you saw a 50ish year old woman being honored for her great wisdom, beauty and achievements? Not often enough, I'm afraid. I spent a great deal of time researching the crone and croning ceremonies and

I looked for ways to honor my fiftieth in a unique way that would set the stage for a celebration that would be meaningful to me.

As I thought about various ways to do that, I began to feel I probably wasn't alone in wanting to celebrate my cronehood, and I could probably make information-gathering about the crone and this rite of passage ceremony a lot easier for like-minded women. That is when I established my company, *Wise Women*™, to be a resource for women who want to learn more about the heritage of the crone and want to acknowledge this cycle of life by holding a croning ceremony. I encourage the aspiring crone to embrace the notion of creating her own personal croning ceremony; where honoring her life's journey, sharing her life's wisdom and experience, and giving clear intention for an extraordinary future is a rite of passage worth celebrating!

My desire to increase awareness of the croning ceremony, and to leave a legacy upon which future crones can build, is the inspiration for this book and the Wise Women website. I sincerely hope that the ideas presented here will inspire, intrigue and delight you. It's as important to me to share my ideas with you as it is to guide you on a path of self-discovery that leads you to appreciating who you are and will become. To crones and wisewomen around the world, let's celebrate!

June Hill, Founder
Wise Women™
www.wisewomenworldwide.com

The Lotus: The Crone

I regard the lotus flower's elegance as similar to an object d'art and analogous to the crone, or wisewoman. Allow me to explain. The sacred lotus flower is known to be an important spiritual symbol in Eastern religions where it represents purity, divine wisdom, and an individual's progress toward the highest state of consciousness. Chinese poets often use the lotus as an inspiration for people to strive through the difficulties of life and show their best side to the outside world no matter how bad things get. To be as a lotus flower, your beauty and light shine through even the murky darkness that lies at the bottom of the pond. I don't know about you, but I've been at the bottom of my murky pond a time or two in my life.

The lotus flower most depicted in art and literature is the white lotus blossom. Its huge, almond-shaped petals form a shallow bowl around a large seed pod. Living in muddy water, the lotus rises every day to produce beautiful, fragrant flowers. Open for only three days, the flower petals then fall quietly back into the water. For quite some time the large, flat seed pod remains and then gradually turns dark and dries. Eventually the large cone shaped pods revert down into the water and will float face down allowing the seeds to germinate and take hold again in the water for the next new show of lotus blossoms.

Did you know that lotus seeds remain active for a very long time? The American Lotus has been known to germinate after a dormant period of 200 years; and recently, lotus seeds from China germinated after 1,200 years! Metaphorically, it speaks to the resiliency of the Triple Goddess archetype (Maiden, Mother, Crone) that rests within the psyches of women. Even throughout our long, patriarchal history, the Goddess archetypal behaviors continued to reside in the very deep recesses of our being.

When I see a lotus blossom, I marvel at the incredible ingenuity of nature. After a hundred million years of evolution, there is still such pristine beauty; such an exquisite design has endured. So it is with the crone, I believe. She has been able to transcend the troubles, challenges and lessons of her spiritual and human experience to become a wiser, more brilliant and beautiful wisewoman.

Chapter 1

------ ◆ ------

YOUR CROWNING ACHIEVEMENT

The Crone

Are you asking "W*hat's a crone?*" and not particularly liking the sound of the word? Well, you're not alone. Many of us feel that way until we better understand what it means to be a crone. I hope that reading this will be the start of a journey that inspires you to learn more about the crone, sometimes known as the wisewoman. I encourage all women to embrace the notion that to be a crone is a crowning achievement in our lives, worth celebrating, and to wear our crowns proudly.

Truth be told, I only became aware of the word "crone" several months before my fiftieth birthday when I began doing research on ceremonies and rituals that honor this rite of passage. Simply speaking, a woman is potentially in the crone phase of her life when she has passed her child bearing years. However, the designation can also refer to a perspective on life or philosophical point of view rather than age or biological change.

I discovered books had been written about the Maiden, Mother and Crone also known as the three aspects of the ancient Triple Goddess archetype. Two books became my Bible: *Crones Don't Whine—Concentrated Wisdom for Juicy Women* and *Archetypes of Older Women—Archetypes in Women over Fifty;* both books written by Dr. Jean Shinoda Bolen, psychiatrist and internationally known Jungian analyst. As I read and reread Bolen's books, I couldn't help but marvel at how eloquently she described the nuances of what I'd been experiencing, thinking, and feeling.

As I learned more about how the behavioral aspects of the goddess archetype figures are activated in the psyches of older women, I was intrigued and excited! At the same time I felt calm, reflective and at peace with how my own life has evolved. I realized that an appreciation of life's experience and spiritual introspection were quite common for a crone. Equally strong are the desires for continuous spiritual growth and for the discovery of one's inner potential. Interestingly, when I mentioned this to most people, their eyes would roll into the back of their heads; and conversely, women that were post-menopausal seemed to understand what I was talking about. It isn't easy to describe, but you know it when it's happening. Nevertheless, these archetypal goddess behaviors seem to emerge whether or not you're aware of them, and believe me; it's much more interesting and amazing when you are aware of them.

You've probably heard the cliché, "Life isn't about the destination but about the journey." For me, these words take on a deeper, more profound meaning in my crone years. To aspire to be a crone is more about a continuous journey of experiences, life long learning and growth, both spiritual and human. The crone is a woman that is gracefully adapting to the process of aging. She quietly inspires others. She is comfortable in her own skin and with her spirituality. Her intuitive and creative powers are pronounced. She has a quiet peacefulness. But what really sets the crone apart is that she embodies a passion to explore meaning in her life; and she exemplifies an unselfish willingness to share her honesty, knowledge, wisdom, love, and compassion.

The Ancient Crone

Before we move on, let's understand how we got here. Allow me to share some perspectives on the history of the crone. In ancient times, c.7000BCE, the words crone, hag and witch were actually *positive* words describing an older woman. Their origins are interesting: *hag* comes from *hagio* meaning *holy*, and *witch* comes from *wit* meaning *wise*. The word *crone* has its origins in the word *crown*; indicative of "wisdom emanating from the head." The ancient custom of placing a crown on the crone's head was and is significant in the croning ceremony, and very symbolic of a crowning achievement in a woman's life.

During these times, the crones, hags and witches were frequently the sages, leaders, midwives and healers in their communities and were revered for their wisdom and knowledge. However, as our history evolved and a patriarchal society took hold, the definitions of the crone, the hag, and the witch were distorted. Unfortunately, these words evolved to have the negative and derogatory connotations that continue today.

I certainly can't predict how other women will internalize the notion of becoming a crone, but the shift in my own perspective was profound when I learned the original definitions of the words. Personally, I believe a shift is occurring and the new crones of today are playing a pivotal role in resurrecting and promoting the more positive perception of the crone. I believe it because we're seeing more and more books being written about women's midlife attitudes and experiences, and that is progress in itself.

The New Crone

Women who have reached their fiftieth birthday milestone over the last two decades and the current wave of baby boomers have had incredible professional and personal opportunities. Now we are exploring our spiritual consciousness through spiritual quests, books, and workshops more than ever before. Additionally, we are seeking spiritual support and affirmation through the formation of spiritually-based women's circles whose mission is to provide support for each other and make a difference in the world. As a result of our work individually and collectively, I believe there will be a massive, positive energy surge from these women over the next several years. It is undeniable; these generations of women have the opportunity to bring back the honored status befitting the crone: she is brilliant, beautiful, extraordinary, and an amazing wisewoman!

Crones, it's up to us to stop in its tracks the negative stereotypes that aging has and redefine it to be the positive experience it is. I like to say it should be about *Pro*-Aging vs. *Anti*-Aging. It should be about *gaining* wisdom vs. *losing* our wits. Rather than turning a blind eye to the attributes of aging, decide to embrace the miracle that is your life!

Chapter 2

THE ROAD TO WOMANHOOD

The Maiden's Menarche

The first time girls are faced with the realization that they are changing is when they experience *menarche,* or their first menstrual period. Some cultures recognize menarche as an important time in a girl's life and celebrate her entry into womanhood, while others view it as an unimportant occurrence, a nuisance, and a "curse." If you think it about, taking the time to honor menarche in a girl's life is probably the first opportunity we have, as women, to introduce the notion of a ceremony that honors womanhood. First, it's a chance to establish a bond between a girl, her mother, and a community of women (aunts, friends, sisters, grandmothers). Secondly, it's an opportunity to introduce the power of a circle of women who can provide guidance, support and comfort; and maybe even help prevent issues that affect young women today, like depression, negative self image and low self-esteem.

Western society tends to overlook menarche; however, increasingly more mothers *want* to celebrate their daughters' first transition to womanhood with the help of a supportive, heartfelt gathering of women and friends. They're beginning to create and hold their own personalized menarche rituals that include music, candles, jewelry, and flowers. I believe it's a sign that the ancient goddess archetypes are re-emerging in those mothers who have realized it's time to again honor this sacred time in a girl's life. Hoorah!

Menarche Rituals from other Cultures

Historically, menarche was celebrated by the ancient Greeks with detailed rituals combining corn with menstrual blood to honor a young girl's future fertility. African, Asian, Middle Eastern and Native American groups are all known to honor menarche with gifts, song, dance and feasts.

The Navajo Kinaalda tradition asks girls to run footraces as a show of strength. Then a cornmeal pudding is shared with the tribe and girls wear special clothing and style their hair like the Navajo Goddess, Changing Woman. The Nootka Indians also thought menarche was a time to test physical strength so girls were taken out to sea and left there. After they swam back to shore, they were cheered by the villagers. Each year, the Mescalero Apaches hold an eight day celebration honoring each girl who began her period that year. The first four days include feasting and dancing and each evening the boys sing about their tribe's history. The next four days are private ceremonies where girls reflect on their rite of passage to womanhood with the women elders in the tribe.

When a Japanese girl gets her first period, the family celebrates by eating red colored rice and beans. In the Ulithi tribe of Micronesia, menarche is called "kufar". A young girl goes to a menstrual house where the women bathe her and recite spells; upon each period she returns to the menstrual house. In the Nigerian Tiv tribe, four lines are cut onto a girl's abdomen and it's believed to make a woman more fertile. In Sri Lanka, in order to predict the girl's future, they note the time and day of her menarch; then an astrologer is contacted to study the stars' alignment at that moment. She's prepared for a ritual bath and washed by the women of the family, then dressed in white and a party ensues where she receives special gifts and money.

Menarche, and then What?

Underlying the question of "then what?" is the question of "why at all?" Why preserve or rebuild the sanctity of rites of passage celebrations anyway? Because rituals and sacred ceremonies have been the foundation, and a vital element, of many cultures for centuries. Some people are doing a better job of preserving or rebuilding the sanctity of rituals than others. It is heartening that, in the case of menarche, some mothers are proactively searching out creative ways to instill a level of reverence and honor around the menarche ritual where previously, there was none.

Rituals are the result of honoring the significance of an event or occasion, generally in a spiritually meaningful way. We have many opportunities to celebrate various occasions but year after year the substance behind our rituals and celebrations gets more and more diluted. An example of this is never as apparent as during the religious celebration, Christmas. Obsessive consumerism and blatant commercialism has replaced the true meaning of the celebration itself.

You can also see the diluted sanctity of celebrations in some time-honored rites of passage or societal life decisions. One example is the "sweet sixteen" or "coming out" party for a young lady, where the significance of this rite of passage to womanhood has morphed into being more about the shopping spree for the perfect dress. Or where there is an opportunity to garner respectability in achieving a rite of passage, instead we choose to pray to the porcelain God or Goddess upon reaching the drinking age. When a woman makes the life altering decision to give life to another human being, the ensuing shower generally revolves around the number of gifts she will receive versus being an opportunity to meaningfully honor that momentous and above all miraculous event. And then there is the "Over the Hill" ritual celebration where black balloons and "humorous" old age jokes and gag gifts ultimately trivializes and minimizes what this rite of passage could be about: honoring one's life journey and achievements in a respectful manner.

There always appears to be a need to introduce disparaging humor or incite embarrassment, which only stands to over-shadow the true meaning of a celebration, particularly in any rite of passage. What I'm trying to say is that the meaningful occasions that occur between menarche and dying; the honor-able, sacred, noteworthy ceremonies for women generally miss the opportunity to imbue within it a sense of spirituality that can manifest the feeling of connectedness to a power that is much bigger than all of us.

A lack of appreciation and awe of our biological phases has permeated western society over hundreds of years. However, we all have the opportunity to appreciate and rebuild the foundation of the spiritual essence of all rituals and ceremo-nies. In particular, those associated with honoring the cycles that women go through as they journey the road to woman-hood. I purposefully say *rebuild* because there was a time in ancient society where the female archetype and her life cycles were revered and respected.

Reintroducing the Croning Ceremony

Ceremonies that honor family or community elders have been done for centuries in many diverse cultures. The Asian culture in particular is known for holding their elders in high esteem. In the Native American tradition, women elders have the opportunity to become part of a Grandmothers Circle and are looked upon for advice and counsel on important issues affecting the tribe. Often being the final decision makers.

More recently, the idea of holding croning ceremonies to celebrate our cronehood is gaining momentum and popularity among older women. As I stated earlier, it's not so much a question of at what age you "become" a crone; it's more about embracing your truth, walking the talk and then acknowledging the designation at a time that feels right to you. Often celebrated around age fifty, ceremonies vary from large or small gatherings of friends to large rituals at women's conferences. Keep in mind that it isn't how you celebrate your cronehood that instills it with meaning, but the fact that you honor this new phase of life as being positive and potentially full of new experiences. An entire lifetime can pass by in the blink of an eye, so this is your chance to give tribute to that life.

Based on my own personal experience with menopause, and in talking with other women, I felt strongly that there were women who were going through this transition and didn't want to bemoan the fact; but instead, were ready to celebrate and honor their lives' journeys and longevity. And while I recognized that menopause wasn't a pleasant experience for many, I still felt that in the end there were many more women who were hopeful and reenergized about their futures, as I was.

Because I felt strongly that women were looking for ways to honor the transition to cronehood, that I established Wise Women™ and determined I would spend my time and energy supporting the continued proliferation of the revered croning ceremony. I know the overwhelming feelings of gratitude I felt when I gathered my dear friends to celebrate my cronehood, and can think of no better way than to help and guide other women in celebrating their lives too.

The croning ceremony that I envision for anyone would reflect the very unique essence of who you are and what you're passionate about. I won't say there are any hard and fast rules for a croning ceremony, except: 1) each person honors the crone in a personal way, often called an offering; either by sharing a reading, music, stories or some other creative way (I share some ideas in this book), and 2) the crone is presented with an emblem that symbolizes her transition to cronehood. Generally it's a crown or decorated wreath that is placed on her head, but the emblem can be whatever you choose, e.g., a piece of jewelry, flower lei, shawl, rattle, drum, or another emblem you feel is appropriate.

While the croning ceremony is a celebration and there should be time to kick up your heels, remember that the focus is the crone and her life's journey. The utmost respect ought to be bestowed her celebration so everyone leaves appreciating the crone and her life's passage.

My Croning Story

For my croning ceremony, I really wanted to honor my close friendships because they've been so important in my life. I wanted to gather together my soul sisters, aka my posse and my cronies. I didn't want the ceremony to be about *me*; I wanted it to be about *us*. It was as simple as that.

I set aside a long weekend to be with my sisters; but a croning ceremony can take place over a week long retreat in a remote location, or it can take place over a weekend, or in a few hours. Obviously, you would tailor your celebration according to your interests, desires, and time constraints.

I wanted to take time to really look at my friends to remember and appreciate why they were my sisters. It was a combination of fellowship, gratitude, love, and reverence—and yes, we had a couple of martinis too. We honored the sisterhood that encircles all women. We affirmed and recognized everyone that was important in shaping who we've become. And finally, we gave clear intention for abundance in all ways, a life full of grace, and a fabulous future.

We had an *Altar of Gratitude* that included photos and memorabilia that reminded us of people and entities that were important in shaping who we've become. We set out flowers and lit candles to help evoke feelings of gratitude and reverence. We spent time talking about the important events and people that represented turning points in our lives. It was as we talked about how we had influenced each other's lives, that I felt an incredible amount of affirmation for why these amazing women were in my life.

In preparation for the croning ceremony, my friends did something unexpected and built a labyrinth in the sand on a beach near my house. I was asked to walk through the labyrinth, symbolizing the journey of my life. Then my friends walked through it symbolizing that I haven't walked alone. When we finished, they placed a fresh flower wreath on my head, symbolizing a crown. In a croning ceremony, the crowning is a gesture that represents and honors the wisdom achieved through one's life experience.

What I am describing here is the croning ceremony that I imagined and made a reality for myself. I wanted it to be unique and meaningful to me, and it was. Undoubtedly, every croning ceremony will be different and unique to the crone—and that's the beauty of a croning ceremony.

When I first started reading about croning ceremonies, my first thought was: I don't want to plan a croning ceremony for myself because that would seem so self serving. Well, one thing I've learned is that we crones *deserve* to think pretty highly of ourselves and if what we want to do is celebrate our lives, then so be it. In addition to feeling good about celebrating our lives with our sisters, we will have created ripples that reach out to other wisewomen whose time has come to celebrate their lives too. And that, my friends, is the start of the swell of crones who finally wear their "crowns" proudly.

I am hopeful that we will bring back the sanctity of all rituals. Ultimately, I sincerely hope that the idea of holding a croning ceremony touches your soul as deeply as it did mine.

"EACH FRIEND REPRESENTS A WORLD IN US, A WORLD POSSIBLY NOT BORN UNTIL THEY ARRIVE, AND IT IS ONLY BY THIS MEETING THAT A NEW WORLD IS BORN."
—Anais Nin

Chapter 3

CELEBRATE YOUR CRONEHOOD

By now I hope you have a better understanding of what it means to aspire to be a crone. Have I given you food for thought and inspired you to hold your own croning ceremony? I hope so. Here are some ideas to get you started, like the invitation. Also in this chapter is an example of a very simple croning ceremony and blessings for you to consider and/or personalize.

The Invitation List—Your Cronies

O.K., so you've decided to hold a croning ceremony. One of the first things you'll think about is "who will I invite?" Not an easy question to answer, but start with who are your soul sisters, who's in your posse, who are your cronies? Who are the women that have been through thick and thin with you? With these women, you've established spiritual bonds. Generally, it occurs when you've experienced something extraordinary together. It might have invoked happiness or sadness, it could've been noteworthy or not, but there was a connection that occurred. You can look back and say, "O.K. that was when I knew we'd be friends forever."

Crones, admit it, haven't you become more selective of whom you let into your circle of friends as you've gotten older? Aren't you more in tune with your posses and recognize the *positive* energy that surrounds you when you get together to talk, reflect, share, and ask for advice? Maybe you've noticed that you're attracting women that really have a *positive* influence on your life; they're candid, supportive, compassionate; and always seem to know the right thing to say (even if it's not what you *want* to hear).

When you look very closely at your life, there will always be a small circle of exceptional women that because of them, your life was transformed. Those, my dear crones, are the women who are your soul sisters—they are in your posse—they are your cronies.

The Invitation

The invitation to your croning ceremony can take many forms. It can be casual or formal, have a special theme or design. Here is a letter that was used as the invitation to a croning ceremony. I used this letter as a template for my own croning invitation. The names have been changed to protect those that graciously allowed me to print their letter.

Dear Cyndi, Marie and Cathy,

You are cordially invited to a celebration of life, originally intended to mark the passage of my 50th birthday, expanded to honor all four of us—our lives, our dreams, our fears and our growth. It will be a circle of four exceptional women, coming together for the first time (perhaps) to share our stories and to celebrate what it means to be a woman in this day and age, moving into our wise woman elder years.

"My friends have made the story of my life."—Helen Keller

You, my dear friends, have made the story of my life. I feel blessed to know each of you and am thrilled that you have agreed to come together for this celebration.

You have all heard much about each other. Most of you have never met, or if you have it was very brief. I'm providing you with a little background about each other…

I met Cyndi in February of 1980 in New York. We were interns together at St. Mary's hospital, neither of us thrilled by the program and the living quarters, we raised hell together and got into all manner of trouble. We have had many far flung adventures over the years, even though we have mellowed considerably. Cyndi has lived in Idaho for the past many years.

I met Marie in December of 1984 when she came to visit her brother Randy for Christmas. Our friendship was slow to start, partly because of the geographical distance and partly because 20 years ago we were very different from each other. Amazing how things change, hmmm? After we lost our designation as sisters-in-law, we simply decided to adopt each other as sisters. After all, we shared her mother for many years. Marie lives in Southern California.

I met Cathy in April of 1987 when she came to my house to buy a mattress that I was selling. (How is that for Divine Intervention?) I knew at once that she was someone I wanted in my life. She lived in Portland at the time so we had a few years to cement our friendship before she returned to Washington, where she currently lives. Cathy has been and continues to be one of the chief sounding boards in my life, always helping me to see things from a broader perspective.

So much for the who…now on to the where…

I have rented a beach house for our celebration for the nights of October 5th, 6th, and 7th. The cost of the lodging is on me, my gift to all of us. (We can all pitch in for groceries and booze.) Check in time is 4:00 so we will leave here about 1:00 to drive over to the coast together. Feel free to arrive and leave when you want.

So much for the details…now on to the celebration…

As I said before, this gathering is really about celebrating our lives. I would love it if we could each be prepared to tell the story of our lives thus far (perhaps no preparation is necessary, but you might want to take some time to think about your childhood years, your rites of passage, the turning points in your lives, people who have had great influence on you, and possibly dreams for the future.) You can take as much or as little time as you wish to tell your story. I would also be thrilled if you could be prepared to lead us through one ritual or ceremony—perhaps something that you have done before or simply something that you feel would be meaningful to do. Again it can be as simple or as elaborate as you wish. I really want this time to be a powerful gathering of spirit; we have so much incredible energy as a collective.

One last thing…Since we are celebrating our births, I would like to create an altar to our mothers for the days that we are at the beach. For good or bad they were and are powerful role models in our lives. Maybe we can talk about the ways we would like to emulate them and the things we choose to do differently than they have. As you know, my mother passed on 17 years ago. Marie's mother passed on much more recently. Cyndi and Cathy's mothers are still alive. Perhaps you can bring something that belonged to your mother or something that your mother gave to you.

These are just ideas that I have. Please feel free to participate in any of these ceremonies or not. If you choose to just sit in the hot tub and walk on the beach for three days, that's fine with me. This time can be healing for all of us.

Lastly and most importantly, I want to thank you for walking beside me in life, for your strength and your support, for your friendship, for putting up with all the parts of me that I am not proud of, for loving me in spite of those parts. Thank you for being my most dear and trusted friends. I am so looking forward to seeing all of you.

With much love,
Chris

Simple Croning Ceremony

Here is a simple, basic croning ceremony for your consideration. Feel free to use any of the ideas in this book or create your own in order to personalize the ceremony. Traditionally, an initiated crone conducts the ceremony, but if that's not possible, anyone that appreciates what it means to be a crone can conduct the ceremony. (You might also consider having a Ceremonialist or Shaman perform the ceremony.) It is a *celebration,* so a feast is an essential element; and there are no rules on eating before or after the ceremony. You'll also find crone blessings to use and/or personalize.

Welcome
Everyone gathers together, ideally in a circle to symbolize the circle of women. Announce the start of the ceremony by sounding a gong, or ringing tingsha bells, playing a singing bowl or chimes, and lighting a candle. Light incense in a bowl to smudge* the space.

Invocation
Invite someone to conduct the invocation (prayer or blessing)
See below for an example.

Presentation of Offerings
Invite each person to share an offering.
See Chapter Four for examples of offerings.

The Transition Emblem Blessing
Bless the emblem that symbolizes the new crone's transition (e.g., crown, necklace, shawl, flowers). An example follows.

The Crone's Initiation
Conduct a blessing for the new crone.
Anoint the new crone with lavender oil and present the emblem to her.

The Crone's Offering
The new crone shares her thoughts upon entering cronehood.

Closing
Invite someone to conduct the closing invocation. An example follows.
End the ceremony by sounding the gong or ringing bells.

* Smudging is the name given to this sacred blessing, a Native American cleansing technique that uses the smoke of dried herbs. Common herbs used are bundles of sage and sweet grass. Smudging asks the spirits of sacred plants to drive away negative energy and to attract positive energy and a sense of balance. It is the psychic equivalent of washing your hands before eating. The notion of purification through smoke is a ritual done around the world in many cultures.

A simple smudging technique can be done by burning incense in a bowl and wafting the smoke around the room. While wafting the smoke say, *"drive away all negativity from our hearts; take away everything unworthy of our attention."* Continue to waft the smoke and imagine it lifting away all negative emotions and energies. Imagine a room cleared of all negativity and now bring in positive energy by saying, *"bring in positive energy for honoring the crone. Help us to be balanced and purify our souls."* Imagine yourselves being surrounded by positive energy, love, wisdom and courage.

Suggestions for Crone Blessings and Initiation

Invocation (to invite, welcome, and honor)
"Greetings of love and a warm welcome to all who gather here today. We come to honor (new crone's name) and to celebrate with her as she enters her crone years, the third stage of womanhood. (New crone's name) has elected this time and place and invited those present to energize and enhance this experience, her right of passage into the realm of the wisewoman.

At this time we invite to join us: the Divine Creator (Whoever that is for you), our Spiritual Guides and Healers, our Angels, and loved ones on other planes of existence. We ask them all to come close and to tenderly mingle their blessed energies with ours. Welcome, all."

Invocation of the Four Directions

This invocation calls in four wisewomen archetypes. In this invocation group yourselves in four sections representing the four directions of North, South, East and West, all facing the center. A lit candle or incense can be placed at the center. Each group speaks in turn from their direction.

"In the East is the rising sun, the dawn of a new day. As we walk the sacred path of life, help us, wisewoman Metis, and goddess of practical and intellectual wisdom. Bring wise counsel and inner wisdom to decisions we make, and can see truth and hope on all paths we choose. Guide our steps and give us courage to express our wisdom with honesty and dignity.

To the South, as we walk the sacred path of life, help us, wisewoman Sophia, and goddess of mystical and spiritual wisdom. Bring intuitive powers that help us understand our path in soulful ways and show us that it is all right to make decisions with our hearts.

To the West is the setting sun. As we walk the sacred path of life, help us, wisewoman Hecate (Hek'a-tē), and goddess of intuitive and psychic wisdom. Help us use our intuition and pay attention to dreams and synchronicities. When we find ourselves at crossroads on our journeys, aid us in listening to the voices of our own intuitive wisdom.

To the North, as we walk the sacred path of life, help us, wisewoman Hestia, and goddess of meditative wisdom. You are the sacred fire within our hearths, and we are drawn to your warmth and find comfort in your presence. Help us to listen to the quiet deep within our souls, and find serenity and comfort in those silences.

(All form a circle and join hands facing the center):

"Goddesses Metis, Sophia, Hecate, and Hestia, thank you all for helping us to know your wisdom. Let Wisdom be our guide."

Blessing the new crone's emblem of initiation

"(New crone's name) has chosen this (identify the emblem) to stand as the emblem of her cronehood during this ceremony. (Take this opportunity to talk about why this emblem was chosen; any special significance it holds.)

At this time we especially call upon Saraswati, the Hindu Goddess of Wisdom, Knowledge, Learning, Creativity, and Rivers to reside with us and place her blessings upon this emblem. Saraswati, your name means literally, Essence of Self; "the one who flows" or "one who moves with the flow of life." You represent to us intelligence, consciousness, cosmic knowledge, creativity, enlightenment, and power. We offer words of gratitude and thanks for your blessing on this emblem and for bestowing these archetypal characteristics upon us. May they become more pronounced in each woman as she crosses over into her crone years."

Crone's Initiation Blessing

"Divine Ones, Goddess Saraswati, Crones, and other honored guests. The time grows near for our beloved sister, (new crone's name), to joyously begin her new life as a crone. Let us be silent for a few moments to join our hearts, minds, and souls with hers as she prepares for this glorious journey. Soon, (new crone's name), will finalize her days as Mother and be reborn as Crone. Soon she will feel a new energy flowing through her veins. She will know she has stepped from an old way of being into a newfound sense of freedom and awareness. We ask that as a new crone you continue to speak your truth, share your wisdom, and become a link between the crones of the ancient past, the recent past, and the crones of the future. Allow me to present our new crone, (insert name), to you."

Closing Ceremony Reading

The following is an ancient reading from the *Wisdom of*

Solomon (an apocryphal Hebrew text written c.100 BCE). It contains text that is attributed to Sophia, Goddess of Wisdom. The language has been modified for modern times.

Wisdom is glorious and never fades away.
She is easily acknowledged by those who love her,
And she is found by those who seek her.
She quickly makes herself known to those who desire her.
Those who seek her shall have no great travail;
For you will find her sitting at your door.
To think therefore upon her is perfection of wisdom,
And those who watch for her shall quickly be without care.
Go about seeking her and make yourself worthy of her,
And she will show herself favorably;
And will meet you in every thought.

"TRUE HAPPINESS IS OF A RETIRED NATURE, AND AN ENEMY TO POMP AND NOISE; IT ARISES, IN THE FIRST PLACE, FROM THE ENJOYMENT OF ONE'S SELF, AND IN THE NEXT FROM THE FRIENDSHIP AND CONVERSATION OF A FEW SELECT COMPANIONS."
—*Joseph Addison*

Chapter 4

CREATIVE WAYS TO CELEBRATE YOUR CRONEHOOD

People have all manner of mental images upon hearing the word "ritual." One of the definitions the word has is: *the performance of actions or procedures in a set, ordered, and ceremonial way.* For the purpose of describing a croning ritual; simply stated, it is a celebration imbued with special meaning or significance. What follows are some creative ways (or offerings) to personalize the croning ceremony ritual.

Activity or Artistic-based Rituals

A ritual is what you make it; it doesn't necessarily have to be something that happens in a church or living room. Your friends might want to get out and be active as part of the celebration. Suggested activities include but certainly not limited to: hiking, bike riding, parasailing, sky diving, repelling down a mountain, mountain climbing, getting pedicures and manicures…you get the idea.

Or your friends might want to do something artistic or creative. How about artistic endeavors like making a collage or painting a mural? Design special artwork and transfer the rendition onto a t-shirt; go to a ceramics shop to make and paint pottery; make jewelry, candles or soaps. The point is that you are doing something as a group that you all enjoy and create a sense of community.

Altars

Altars are traditionally a place of honor in the home and help to connect you to important people or entities in your life. For an *Altar of Gratitude* at your croning ceremony, have everyone bring items that inspire gratitude in their lives like pictures, mementos, jewelry from someone, crystals, rocks, or figurines—anything that holds special memories. Make the alter really special with lit candles, burning incense and/or a beautiful bouquet of flowers.

An *Altar to the Crone* is also a beautiful way to honor her. Ask everyone to bring items that remind them of the crone. As part of the croning ceremony, ask everyone to share their stories about the items they've brought.

Anointing the Crone

The word *anoint* is derived from the Old French word *enoint*, or "smeared on." Originally it referred to oil smeared on for medicinal purposes. The anointing process has evolved over centuries and is still used ritually by many religions and cultures for baptisms, coronations, or spiritual and religious ceremonies. Some ceremonial anointing oil recipes are very closely guarded secrets and once consecrated, are protected by ceremonial law and only to be used in specific ceremonies.

Anointing the crone is a way to invite her into cronehood

and generally is combined with presenting the transition emblem. If you chose to include this in the ceremony, many companies produce bottled spray infusions, sometimes known as Aura Sprays. The sprays are made with oils or water infused with various essential oils or flower essences. At the appropriate time in the ceremony, gently spray an arc over and around the crone (avoid the eyes). Another easy way to anoint the crone is simply put a dot of an essential oil on the crone's forehead. Lavender, known for its soothing qualities is commonly used in rituals. Please be mindful of any possible allergies and manufacturer's safety precautions.

Ceremonialists or Shamans

Ceremonialists or Shamans have knowledge and experience in many old traditions, rituals, and ceremonies from many cultures that honor rites of passage through music, chants, song or special invocations. They can work with you to create a ceremony that will be meaningful to you. Ceremonialists and Shamans often have websites that you can find on the internet, some may advertise in newspapers, magazines, or have information on community boards in public places like health food stores, houses of worship, or spiritual and metaphysical shops.

Crone Treasure Chest

The treasure chest or a special beautiful box can be used to symbolically hold the spiritual space for items that are important to the crone and others participating in the ceremony. Ask everyone to think about people, things or entities that they are grateful for in their lives. Have them write it down on paper and place it in the treasure chest. If the box is large enough, have people bring mementos that remind them of important people or entities and place them in the box. A special box could also be used as the transition emblem. During the croning ceremony the treasure chest or sacred box would be honored through a blessing or prayer and presented to the crone.

Fire Ceremony

This ritual reminds me of a favorite, old Chinese proverb, *"My barn having burned to the ground, I can now see the moon."* Fire ceremonies have been used for centuries in diverse cultures to manifest healing, purify the spirit, mind and body. For the purpose of a croning ceremony, the fire ceremony can be used to resolve or release any old feelings, issues, or attitudes. And then invite new attitudes of cronehood to permeate your being and to be a source of inspiration and wisdom for new and upcoming crones.

Here's how: build a fire in a safe place like a kettle BBQ, beach fire pit, or wood burning fireplace. Give each person two pieces of paper. On one piece write, "Resolve or Release" and the other, "Invite In"; then ask everyone to focus on the attitudes they want to "release" or "invite" and write them down. Have everyone stand near the fire and one at time; place their "release" note in the fire while saying: *"We come to the fire with gratitude for its healing power; we feel the healing power in our bodies, minds, and spirits; we release and resolve all issues that linger."* Then place the "invite" note into the fire while saying: *"We come to the fire with gratitude for all it provides; we feel its warmth, magic, and power to deliver our wishes under grace and in a perfect way."* Placing something in the fire is symbolic of giving way to the Universe and doesn't necessarily have to be pieces of paper. Commonly used are cuttings from a tree that are decorated and spiritually imbued. Ultimately, this is a celebration and everyone is encouraged to open their hearts, minds and souls to the energies of the fire ceremony.

Gift Giving

While a croning ceremony is all about the crone and offerings or gifts are usually given to her, I have often suggested
that the crone reciprocate by presenting gifts to her friends.
Receiving a gift from the crone shows her love and affection
in a very unique and memorable way. Handmade gifts are, of
course, also a nice option if the crone has crafty, artistic abilities. If she has chosen to do this, you might ask her to make
a special presentation and share how she's been influenced by
her friends. For my croning I made Chinese coin and amethyst
pendants, strung with silk cord. My friends loved their personalized gifts; they were unique, and my friends will remember
me when they wear them.

Labyrinth

An ancient meditation technique, the labyrinth, is sometimes known as a "spiritual tool" that predates Christianity
and was widely used in Christian spirituality until the 16th cen-
tury. There are historical accounts of the labyrinth and its in-
clusion in medieval cathedrals, particularly the one at Chartres
in France.

This takes some preparation and might require some strong
people to put together depending on what medium you use,
but it's a wonderful way to make the ceremony unique and
special. Create a labyrinth out of large stones, luminaries, large
shells or anything that would indicate a path or design on the
ground. Place your items in a pattern that allows enough room
for a pathway. If you're lucky enough to be near or on a beach,
use a rake to create a meandering path in the sand. An easy
labyrinth that we used at my croning ceremony was a contem-

porary variation, called a Vesica Triangle. More information on labyrinths can be found at www.labyrinthsociety.org.

At the start of the croning ceremony, have the crone enter the labyrinth and slowly walk the path, signifying the journey of her life. As the crone completes the labyrinth, symbolically, she's come through the trials of life and now enters her crone phase. Have each person walk the labyrinth signifying that the crone will not walk alone. When everyone is finished walking the labyrinth, it's a good time to present the crone with her transition emblem.

Laugh Out Loud!

Crone passion #1: we love good, deep belly laughs! By the time we reach cronehood, finding the humor in life comes naturally and the ability to laugh at ourselves gets easier. What a great way to set the stage for a laugh-out-loud circle of women by asking everyone to come with some good jokes, yarns, or stories. Ask everyone to bring stories about their lives, the crone, or an event that occurred with the crone that inspired the best, biggest belly laugh of their lives. Have fun with this one!

Music, Chants, Songs, and the Drumming Circle

People all over the world get together and harmonize with each other through music, songs, chants or percussion. For a croning ceremony, use the power of music and rhythm to unite the women's circle. If you're lucky enough to have someone in your circle with musical talent, like playing the piano, dedicate a beautiful song (perhaps the crone's favorite) to the crone. Or have someone compose a song to the crone and sing it together. Drumming circles and the rhythm of music are a popular way to bond with people and community. If exploring your rhythmical spirituality through a drumming circle is of interest, books and products are available that can help you explore this powerful experience. Native American and African drums and rattles are often available at holistic health fairs and on the internet.

Portrait of the Crone

Here's a fun, artistic way for everyone to share their thoughts and feelings about the crone through their own creative, artistic renditions. Give everyone a box of crayons or big colorful markers and a big piece of artist's paper or butcher's meat wrapping paper (flip chart paper also works). Ask each person to think about the crone and then draw a picture. Everyone gets about thirty minutes to go somewhere private to draw their pictures and when everyone comes back together, have them share their drawings. As a lasting memory of the ceremony, the crone keeps all the pictures and maybe even has them framed!

Photo Album or Memory Book

An album or memory book with photographs from the crone's life is a nice, memorable keepsake to present. Put this together by asking everyone to bring their favorite photograph(s) of the crone; it might be from a memorable trip taken together. During the ceremony, the album is passed around and each person shares her story about the photograph(s).

Put on a Play!

No doubt you've seen Mickey Rooney say to Judy Garland in any number of movies they made together, "hey, let's put on a show!" Many years ago I attended a 40th birthday party where friends created a play that reflected the idiosyncrasies and characterizations of the birthday girl. Complete with costumes, wigs, and things that brought out the persona of our friend, we produced several vignettes that chronicled her life. There was a vignette about her distinct clothing style which at that time leggings and big tops was the fashion. The tribute was creative, funny, poignant, and had us all crying and rolling in the aisles (or living room). What an original, entertaining way to honor the crone. Someone that has technical abilities could even tape the show and produce a DVD that is given to everyone as a lasting memory.

Ribbon Braiding Ceremony

This tradition is a very old wedding tradition where the couple braids three strands of ribbon to symbolize the unification of the couple. It can be easily modified for the croning ceremony where it symbolizes the spirit and friendship of the women's circle. In this ceremony there are long, different colored ribbons, strands or ropes. You will need a minimum of three strands for a braid. Cut each strand to approximately four or five feet long. Depending on the number of people in the group you might have more than one person hold a strand or you may make more than one braid. Have everyone braid their strands in a cooperative effort that symbolizes the mutual commitment that you will always support each other with spirit and friendship. The final braid(s) are blessed and draped over the crone's shoulders. Or you can initially cut the strands long enough so that the finished braid forms one circle around everyone and symbolizes your united circle of wise-women. Or connect several braids end to end to form one long braid around the circle.

Sand Ceremony

In the ancient Hawaiian tradition, a sand ceremony is used to symbolically unite couples in marriage by combining the sand from beneath their feet in a beautiful shell. The metaphor being that the combined sand from beneath their feet symbolizes the lasting legacy of their marriage.

The sand ceremony can be modified for the croning ceremony by giving the crone a beautiful shell and have her pass it around so each person can put sand from beneath their feet into the shell. After it's gone around to each person, perform a blessing and place it in the middle of the circle. The sand in the shell symbolizes the unity of the women's circle and their lasting friendships.

For a variation on this if you're not near a beach, you can often purchase colored sand at a craft store. Purchase small bags of different colored sand for each participant and the crone. Buy small bud vases for each person and pour each color into its own vase. Buy a separate beautiful bottle, like a heart-shaped bottle with a top, ensuring it's big enough to hold all the sand. During the ceremony, each person will pour her vase of sand into the heart-shaped bottle one at a time to create a colorful layered pattern. Again, this symbolizes the unity of the women's circle and also creates a unique sand design in the bottle for the crone to keep. You don't have to use sand; you can also use rice, seeds, beans, herbs, colored bath salts, or other pourable materials that will create layers.

The Talking Stick and Talking Stone

In the Native North American tradition the talking stick is essential to special council meetings or gatherings. It allows each member to present their point of view without interruption. Here's how: everyone sits in a circle and the talking stick is passed around and, in turn, each person is allowed to share their truth. Out of respect for the speaker, only those holding the talking stick are allowed to speak. If the speaker would like to ask a question of someone, a feather is passed to that person and is given permission to answer the query. The feather is called an Answering Feather and is generally an eagle feather which signifies truth.

The talking stick is a ceremonial item that is beautifully decorated to show the individual Chief or elder's accomplishments and spirituality. Eagle feathers, cured leather, crystals or beads are typically used. The type of tree used in making a talking stick is also symbolic. For example; Maple represents gentleness, Elm is used for wisdom, Oak for strength, Cherry for expression, high emotion, or love, and fruit woods represent abundance.

Ornamentation of the talking stick has meaning. In the Lakotah tradition, red is for life, yellow is for knowledge, blue is for prayer and wisdom, white is for spirit, purple is for healing, orange is for feeling kinship with all living things, and black is for clarity and focus.

In keeping with the Native American tradition, the crone would be responsible for decorating her own talking stick by finding a large stick or cutting off a tree or bush. Ideas to decorate her talking stick include shells, crystals, beads, feathers, and anything that represents the crone's accomplishments or spirituality. Ultimately, what it looks like is less important than the importance imbued in its making.

Also used for the purpose of showing respect to the speaker, is a talking stone. Stones engraved with words of wisdom or hand carved figurines out of soapstone or alabaster can often be found in local artist's galleries. During the croning ceremony, have everyone sit in a circle. The crone will hand the "talking emblem" to each person so she is allowed to speak her truth without interruption, share stories, and express feelings about the crone. After the ceremony, the emblem could be used by the crone anytime the art of communication is needed.

Transition Emblem—the Crone's "Crowning"

The crone's initiation is very significant in the croning ceremony and symbolizes her passage into the wisewoman years. As I explained earlier, the word *crone* is derived from the word *crown* indicating "wisdom emanating from the head." The presentation of an emblem generally culminates the ceremony. The emblem itself can take many forms, but most common is a crown or headpiece that the crone wears on her head. Other ideas include a piece of jewelry like a necklace, a shawl or cloak, a drum or rattle, or a special box. Of course you could have a beautiful crown headpiece plus give an emblem or gift to the crone.

In the Hawaiian tradition, fresh flower leis and, specifically, haku leis (flower head piece or wreath) are given to people of honor at special occasions like birthdays, graduations, or weddings. Ordering fresh flower and haku leis is a nice gesture and can be preordered and shipped direct from Hawaii. Local florists can also create a flower head piece or lei for you.

A small wreath crown can also be made from silk flowers and is an everlasting memory. It can be made by purchasing a small grapevine wreath at a crafts store and embellishing it with beads, flowers, shells, or with little items that represent or are important to the crone.

Tributes to the Crone

A special tribute to the crone can be presented by someone that knows the crone well or shared experiences with her that create a legacy upon which the group can honor and appreciate. This is similar to a eulogy, but instead it's a "living" tribute that celebrates her life. If someone has technical abilities, a video or slide presentation complete with a collage of photographs and a musical overlay is a wonderful way to make it a lasting, special tribute.

Unity Candles

Have everyone sit in a circle with their own candle. The idea here is that each person lights her candle and shares her thoughts, memories or stories about the crone. Small votive candles are good for this; as each person begins her story, she lights her candle and places it in the center of the group on a table or other flat surface. Or floating candles can be used beautifully; as each person lights her candle, she places it in a large bowl of water that sits in the middle of the group. The effect of the lit, floating candles is lovely. Another idea to symbolize unity is for everyone to have a lit candle and have the group all together light the crone's candle.

These are just a sampling of ideas; and I hope I've inspired many more ideas in you, my dear crone. I think you will see a common thread in the examples I've presented: spirituality, unity, accord, fun, camaraderie, friendship, and support; which are all representative of a women's circle.

AFTERTHOUGHT

Please allow me one final pontification. As I wrote this book, always on my mind was the sisterhood of which we are all a part. We all have our own circle of women friends, our sisterhood, our circle of influence, our people, or our tribe. And while there are millions of women that are outside our sphere of direct influence, virtually we are all one. I am never struck more, or feel our "oneness" more, than when I see a "sister" on the national stage and she is sharing her triumph, sharing her challenge, or she is suffering. It's during these times that, even though I'm not in her circle, I'm still compelled to internalize the joy of her triumph, give her strength to meet the challenge, and feel compassion for her suffering as if it were my own.

Having grown up an only child, people always ask me, *"Didn't you miss having brothers and sisters?"* My answer is always the same, *"no."* Not having a circle of siblings made me appreciate the fact that my circle of girlfriends would always be important in my life and I would need to nurture those friendships. I always knew that I would be responsible for creating my own circle of women and friends, and I was O.K. with that.

While I was growing up I spent the majority of my youth at my best friend Terry's house. Her family was Bolivian and embodied the term "extended family", so they never made me feel that I wasn't part of their family. The concept of the women's circle ritual was first introduced to me at Terry's house when I was in high school. More often than not, you'd find me, Terry, her sister Linda, their mother, aunts, cousins, and grandmothers around the kitchen table where we sat for *hours*. Around that table we shared cups of coffee with hot milk (the latte of the 70's), we played cards, we polished our nails, the women smoked, the grandmothers cooked and baked, and overarching everything was conversation and laughter—and boy did we have some laughs around that table. People would come and go all day long but you could always be certain to find someone to sit with at that kitchen table. This kitchen table community of girls and women was a safe place where we could all tell our stories and have them be heard and acknowledged. Of course, there were men and boys that would come around, but it was the women that really owned that table.

Thinking back on those times, I still feel the authenticity of that sisterhood even after thirty-five years. It was my first introduction to the proverbial women's circle and I always found that human connection around the kitchen table to be spiritual and affecting. It was a period in my life that I'll never forget, and I'll be eternally grateful to the Williamson family.

I am disheartened to think about the extinction of the kitchen table community. When I look around today, who has time to build one when kids are triple booked with extracurricular activities, parents are driving kids all over the countryside, fifty hour workweeks are the new forty hour workweeks, and quality time with family is rare.

In many ways, the kitchen table community is the precursor to the women's circle. Unfortunately for many, the kitchen table is never played out. So if young girls lack the human and spiritual connection that ultimately forms within a circle of women, will they ever understand and connect to its power? As the advent of technology moves us further away from the visceral, spiritual, and human connection, I contend that younger girls will find it hard to understand, much less experience, the one-on-one power of the kitchen table community with their women elders. I'm afraid it'll only get off the endangered list when it becomes a priority of the family matriarchs.

Having said that; I do, however, believe that the crones of today are again realizing the power of the women's circle as more and more are forming thanks to encouragement from Dr. Jean Shinoda Bolen in her book, *The Millionth Circle— How to Change Ourselves and the World*. Today's crones have a tremendous opportunity to set the stage for the proliferation of the wisewomen circles, and in so doing, will act as role models for the crones-in-waiting who, hopefully, will realize the power of the kitchen table community again. I have a dream...wouldn't it be great if we started seeing young girls unplug from their music players and walk away from their televisions and computers because they'd rather sit around the kitchen table to hear and share stories with their moms, sisters, aunts, grandmothers and friends? Wow...

So as you acknowledge your divine cronehood, share your wisdom and knowledge with your circles of women in all its forms. Gather with other crones and crones-in-waiting to make a lasting difference around the kitchen table and ultimately around the world.

With love to you on your journey,

June

FINAL THOUGHT

Share your Ideas and Stories

It is my sincere hope and desire that you are inspired to hold your own unique croning ceremonies. I invite you to share your stories with me so together we can build a collection of croning stories and ideas to share with other wisewomen in a future publication.

It is preferred that all submissions are sent via the website. If you don't have access to the internet, please send or fax your submissions to:

Wise Women
P.O. Box 461556
Escondido, CA 92046
Fax: 760-294-9361
Website: www.wisewomenworldwide.com

Stories should be typed on plain white 8½ x 11 inch paper, in 12-pt Times New Roman font. Include author's contact information: name, address, and phone number. No anonymous submissions please. Stories should be limited to a maximum of 1200 words. Mail your submission in a flat, 9x12 envelope if possible. Send only one copy. Submissions (including photos or other media) will not be returned, so please don't send originals.

To all crones and wisewomen that take the time to write,

thank you. In hearing how you have honored yourselves and how your friends have honored you, I will know that perhaps I influenced that human and spiritual connection in some small way.

ABOUT THE AUTHOR

June Hill's life journey includes being an active participant in corporate America for twenty-five years as a loyal worker bee. In a gutsy maneuver; she walked away from her cubicle in her late 40's, sold everything, left her friends and family behind, and moved to Hawaii to begin her midlife renaissance. After a great deal of soul searching and introspection, she realized her desire to follow her family's history of entrepreneurialism.

To forge awareness and remove the mystery of the crone and croning ceremonies became the inspiration for her first book, *Midlife Musings: Creative Croning Ceremonies,* and then established her company, *Wise Women*™. She assists women who want to hold croning ceremonies and carries a line of Wise Women™ gifts which are available through the website. She currently lives in Southern California where she enjoys walking on the beach with her Pembroke corgi, Sophie.

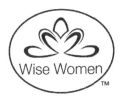

www.wisewomenworldwide.com

NOTES

NOTES

NOTES

NOTES

NOTES

NOTES

Made in the USA
Las Vegas, NV
16 October 2022